LEAKY GUT COOKBOOK

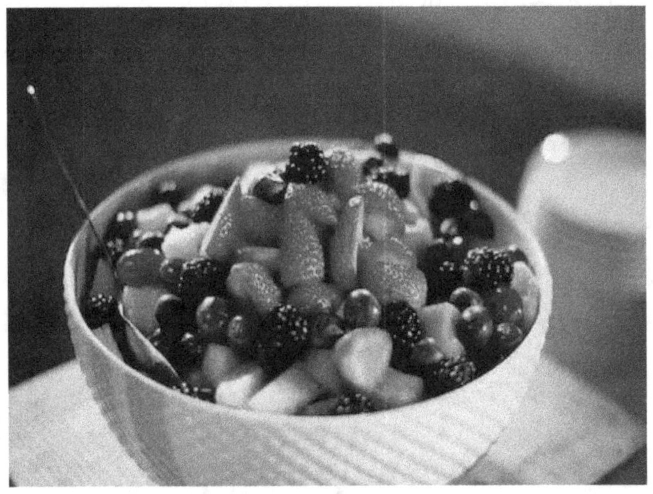

DR. JESSICA SMITH

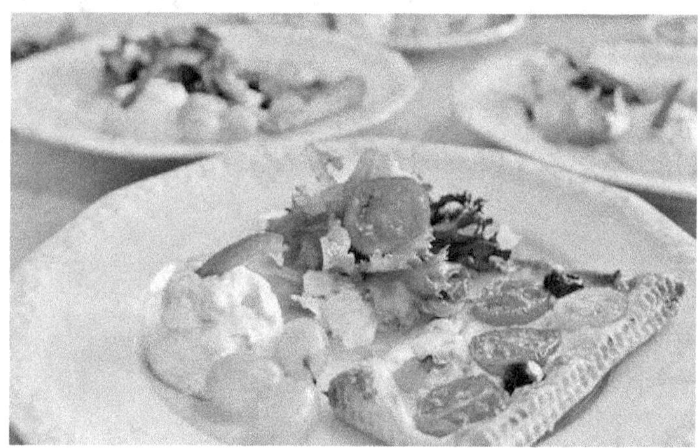

TABLE OF CONTENT

INTRODUCTION TO LEAKY GUT

In recent years, the concept of "leaky gut" has gained prominence as a potential culprit behind a myriad of health issues. This phenomenon, scientifically known as increased intestinal permeability, refers to a condition where the lining of the gastrointestinal tract becomes compromised, allowing undigested food particles, toxins, and bacteria to leak into the bloodstream.

While the medical community is still exploring the intricacies of this condition, there is a growing acknowledgment of its possible connections to various health problems.

At its core, the intestinal lining serves as a formidable barrier, selectively allowing nutrients to pass through while preventing harmful substances from entering the bloodstream.

However, when this barrier is compromised, it sets the stage for a cascade of potential health challenges. The causes of a leaky gut are diverse, ranging from a poor diet and chronic stress to imbalances in the gut microbiome.

Understanding the signs and symptoms of a leaky gut is crucial for early detection and intervention. Individuals experiencing digestive issues, chronic fatigue, autoimmune conditions, and even skin problems may find that their symptoms trace back to an underlying issue of intestinal permeability.

In this journey of exploration, we delve into the fundamentals of leaky gut, unraveling the complexities that surround its origins and manifestations.

From the crucial role of the gut microbiome to the impact of dietary choices, each aspect contributes to the intricate web of factors influencing gut health.

By gaining a deeper understanding of leaky gut, we equip ourselves with the knowledge needed to make informed lifestyle choices and embark on a path toward healing and gut restoration.

CHAPTER ONE

Definition and Basics

Leaky gut, also known as intestinal permeability, is a condition that fundamentally alters the dynamics of the gastrointestinal system. At its essence, the intestines possess a selectively permeable lining that regulates the passage of substances from the digestive tract into the bloodstream.

In a healthy state, this barrier acts as a vigilant gatekeeper, allowing essential nutrients to be absorbed while blocking the entry of harmful substances. However, when the integrity of this barrier is compromised, the stage is set for what is commonly referred to as a "leaky gut."

The term "leaky gut" vividly describes the situation where the tight junctions between the cells of the intestinal lining become more permeable than usual.

This heightened permeability allows undigested food particles, toxins, and bacteria to leak through and enter the bloodstream. As these foreign entities breach the gut barrier, the immune system may mount an inflammatory response, potentially contributing to a range of health issues.

Understanding the basics of a leaky gut involves recognizing the factors that can contribute to its development. Poor dietary choices, chronic stress, infections, and imbalances in the gut microbiome are among the various culprits that can compromise the intestinal barrier. Moreover, certain medications and environmental factors may also play a role in exacerbating this condition.

To address the complexities of leaky gut, it becomes imperative to comprehend not only the anatomical changes occurring within the gastrointestinal tract but also the diverse array of factors that influence its development.

By grasping the definition and basics of leaky gut, individuals gain insight into the intricate interplay between lifestyle, gut health, and overall well-being, laying the groundwork for informed and proactive health management.

Causes and Risk Factors

Unraveling the intricate web of causes and risk factors behind a leaky gut is crucial for understanding the multifaceted nature of this condition. While the exact etiology remains a subject of ongoing research, several factors have been identified as potential contributors to the development of increased intestinal permeability.

One primary factor is dietary choices. Consuming a diet high in processed foods, refined sugars, and lacking in fiber can disrupt the delicate balance of the gut microbiome. This imbalance, known as dysbiosis, can compromise the integrity of the intestinal lining, paving the way for a leaky gut.

Gluten, a protein found in wheat and other grains, has also been implicated in increasing gut permeability in susceptible individuals.

Chronic stress stands out as another significant player in the realm of leaky gut. Stress activates the body's "fight or flight" response, releasing hormones that can impact the gut's functionality. Prolonged stress may lead to inflammation and alterations in gut permeability, exacerbating the risk of a leaky gut.

Infections, both acute and chronic, can also contribute to intestinal permeability. Pathogenic bacteria and certain parasites have been linked to disruptions in the gut barrier.

Additionally, the use of nonsteroidal anti-inflammatory drugs (NSAIDs) and certain medications, such as antibiotics, may play a role in compromising gut health.

Genetic predispositions and autoimmune conditions further heighten the risk of developing a leaky gut. Individuals with a family history of gastrointestinal issues or autoimmune diseases may be more susceptible to alterations in gut permeability.

By acknowledging and understanding these diverse causes and risk factors, individuals can make informed lifestyle choices to support gut health and reduce the likelihood of a leaky gut, underscoring the importance of a holistic approach to well-being.

Signs and Symptoms

Detecting a leaky gut involves paying close attention to a spectrum of signs and symptoms that can manifest throughout the body.

While these indicators may vary among individuals, certain common themes emerge, providing valuable insights into the potential presence of increased intestinal permeability.

Digestive disturbances often take center stage, with symptoms such as chronic diarrhea, constipation, bloating, and abdominal pain signaling possible gut dysfunction. Individuals may also experience fluctuations in weight, as nutrient absorption becomes compromised in the presence of a leaky gut.

Beyond the digestive realm, systemic symptoms may surface. Fatigue, often chronic and unexplained, can be an early indicator of a leaky gut's impact on overall health. Joint pain, headaches, and skin issues like rashes or acne may also arise.

The connection between the gut and the skin, often referred to as the gut-skin axis, underscores the far-reaching consequences of intestinal permeability.

Immune system responses play a pivotal role in leaky gut manifestations. Frequent infections, allergies, and sensitivities to certain foods may indicate an overactive immune response triggered by the influx of undigested particles into the bloodstream. Mental health c an be affected as well, with symptoms like mood swings, anxiety, and difficulty concentrating potentially linked to gut-brain axis disturbances associated with a leaky gut.

Recognizing these signs and symptoms prompts individuals to seek medical evaluation and explore lifestyle changes that support gut health. It also underscores the interconnectedness of various bodily systems, emphasizing the importance of a holistic approach to well-being. A

s the understanding of leaky gut evolves, vigilance in identifying and addressing these signs becomes instrumental in fostering overall health and resilience.

The Gut Microbiome

Located in the intricacies of the gastrointestinal tract lies a community of microorganisms collectively known as the gut microbiome.

This complex ecosystem, comprised of bacteria, viruses, fungi, and other microbes, plays a pivotal role in maintaining the delicate balance of the digestive system and influencing broader aspects of human health.

At its core, the gut microbiome contributes to digestion and nutrient absorption, aiding in the breakdown of complex carbohydrates and synthesizing certain vitamins.

Beyond these essential functions, it acts as a guardian of the intestinal barrier, helping to fortify its integrity and defend against potential breaches that could lead to a leaky gut.

The symbiotic relationship between the host and the microbiome is a dynamic dance of mutual benefit. The microbiome helps educate the immune system, training it to distinguish between friend and foe. Conversely, the host provides a nourishing environment for these microorganisms to thrive.

Imbalances in the gut microbiome, known as dysbiosis, have been linked to a variety of health issues, including inflammatory bowel diseases, allergies, and metabolic disorders.

Disruptions in this delicate microbial equilibrium can contribute to increased intestinal permeability, underlining the profound impact of the gut microbiome on gut health.

Maintaining a healthy gut microbiome involves a multifaceted approach. Dietary choices rich in fiber, fermented foods, and prebiotics nourish beneficial microbes. Antibiotic use, stress management, and avoidance of excessive hygiene practices also play roles in preserving microbial diversity.

As research continues to unravel the mysteries of the gut microbiome, it becomes increasingly evident that fostering a harmonious relationship with these microscopic inhabitants is key to promoting not only digestive wellness but also the broader symphony of human health.

The Importance of a Healthy Microbiome

Within the intricate landscape of the human body, the microbiome emerges as a crucial player, exerting a profound influence on overall health and well being.

Comprising trillions of microorganisms, including bacteria, viruses, and fungi, the microbiome forms a dynamic ecosystem primarily located in the gastrointestinal tract. The importance of maintaining a healthy microbiome extends far beyond digestive processes, encompassing a myriad of physiological functions essential for human vitality.

One of the pivotal roles of a healthy microbiome is its contribution to digestion and nutrient absorption. Beneficial bacteria assist in breaking down complex carbohydrates, producing enzymes that facilitate the extraction of essential nutrients from food.

This symbiotic relationship enhances the efficiency of the digestive system, ensuring that the body receives the nutrients it needs for optimal functioning.

Equally significant is the microbiome's impact on the immune system. A diverse and balanced microbial community helps educate the immune system, teaching it to recognize and respond appropriately to potential threats. This immune training is integral to maintaining a vigilant defense against pathogens while preventing unnecessary inflammatory responses.

Moreover, the microbiome acts as a guardian of the gut barrier, playing a vital role in preventing the occurrence of a leaky gut. A healthy balance of microbes contributes to the integrity of the intestinal lining, fortifying it against the intrusion of harmful substances into the bloodstream.

This protective function is key to averting systemic inflammation and safeguarding against various health issues.

Recent scientific discoveries link the microbiome not only to digestive and immune health but also to mental well-being, metabolic function, and even chronic diseases.

As our understanding of the microbiome deepens, nurturing its diversity and balance emerges as a cornerstone of preventive healthcare, emphasizing the profound impact that these microscopic allies wield in shaping our overall health trajectory.

Imbalance and Leaky Gut

The delicate equilibrium of the gut microbiome, when disrupted, can set the stage for the development of a leaky gut. Imbalance within this microbial community, referred to as dysbiosis, occurs when there is a disproportionate ratio of beneficial to harmful microorganisms.

Dysbiosis is a critical factor in the intricate interplay leading to increased intestinal permeability. Beneficial bacteria in the gut contributes to the maintenance of the intestinal barrier's integrity. They produce substances that nourish the cells lining the gut, promote tight junctions between these cells, and help modulate the immune system. When dysbiosis occurs, harmful microbes may proliferate, leading to a breakdown of this protective barrier.

In a state of imbalance, the gut microbiome may lose its diversity, and the delicate ecosystem becomes disrupted. This can result from various factors, including a poor diet rich in processed foods and low in fiber, overuse of antibiotics, chronic stress, and environmental exposures.

As dysbiosis takes root, the gut barrier becomes more susceptible to compromise. The imbalance may trigger inflammation and immune responses, contributing to the permeability of the intestinal lining.

Harmful substances, such as undigested food particles and toxins, can then pass through the compromised barrier and enter the bloodstream, eliciting systemic reactions.

Addressing imbalance is a pivotal aspect of leaky gut prevention and management. Restoring a healthy balance in the gut microbiome involves adopting a holistic approach, including dietary changes that support beneficial microbes, reducing stress, and avoiding unnecessary antibiotic use.

Understanding the intricate relationship between microbial balance and gut health underscores the significance of maintaining harmony within this microbial community to safeguard against the potential consequences of a leaky gut.

Strategies for Microbiome Health

Nurturing a thriving and balanced gut microbiome is essential for overall well-being, and adopting proactive strategies can contribute significantly to its health.

These strategies encompass lifestyle choices, dietary habits, and mindful practices aimed at fostering a diverse and resilient microbial community within the gastrointestinal tract.

Dietary Diversity:

A diverse diet rich in fiber, fruits, vegetables, and fermented foods provides essential nutrients that support the growth of beneficial bacteria.

These microbes, in turn, contribute to the fermentation of dietary fibers, producing short-chain fatty acids that nourish the cells lining the gut.

Prebiotics and Probiotics:

Introducing prebiotic-rich foods, such as garlic, onions, and bananas, supports the growth of beneficial bacteria. Probiotics, found in fermented foods like yogurt and kefir, can directly introduce live beneficial bacteria into the gut, enhancing microbial diversity.

Limiting Antibiotic Use:

Antibiotics, while essential in treating infections, can disrupt the balance of the gut microbiome. Responsible and targeted antibiotic use, coupled with strategies to restore the microbiome afterward, helps mitigate the potential negative effects.

Stress Management:

Chronic stress can adversely impact the gut microbiome. Practices like mindfulness meditation, deep breathing exercises, and regular physical activity contribute not only to stress reduction but also to a healthier gut environment.

Adequate Sleep:

Quality sleep is crucial for overall health, including the well-being of the gut microbiome.

Establishing consistent sleep patterns supports the circadian rhythms that influence microbial activity in the gut.

Avoiding Overly Hygienic Practices:

Excessive use of antibacterial soaps and a hyper-hygienic lifestyle may strip the environment of beneficial microbes. Embracing a more balanced approach to hygiene preserves microbial diversity.

These strategies collectively promote a resilient and balanced gut microbiome, contributing not only to digestive health but also to systemic well-being.

As our understanding of the microbiome continues to evolve, these proactive measures empower individuals to take an active role in cultivating and preserving a flourishing microbial community within.

CHAPTER TWO

The Link Between Diet and Leaky Gut

Diet plays a pivotal role in the delicate balance between gut health and the development of a leaky gut. The choices we make in terms of what we eat can significantly influence the integrity of the intestinal barrier and the overall health of the gastrointestinal tract.

Processed Foods and Sugar:

A diet high in processed foods and refined sugars is a common contributor to increased intestinal permeability. These foods may promote the growth of harmful bacteria while diminishing the presence of beneficial microbes, disrupting the balance critical for a healthy gut.

Gluten and Certain Proteins:

Gluten, found in wheat and other grains, has been implicated in some cases of leaky gut. Additionally, certain proteins derived from dairy and other sources may contribute to gut inflammation and compromise the integrity of the intestinal lining in susceptible individuals.

Lack of Fiber:

Inadequate fiber intake can deprive beneficial bacteria of their preferred energy source, hindering their growth. Fiber-rich foods, such as fruits, vegetables, and whole grains, support the production of short-chain fatty acids that nourish the cells lining the gut and help maintain tight junctions.

Nutrient Deficiencies:

A diet lacking essential nutrients, including vitamins and minerals, can impair the repair and regeneration of the gut lining. Adequate nutrition is crucial for sustaining the cells that form the protective barrier.

Pro-Inflammatory Foods:

Certain foods, such as those high in saturated fats and artificial additives, may trigger inflammation in the gut. Chronic inflammation can compromise the integrity of the intestinal lining and contribute to leaky gut development.

Conversely, adopting an anti-inflammatory and gut-friendly diet rich in diverse, whole foods can contribute to a healthier intestinal environment. Prioritizing nutrient-dense meals, incorporating probiotic-rich foods, and minimizing the consumption of potential inflammatory triggers form the cornerstone of dietary strategies to support gut health and reduce the risk of a leaky gut.

The Impact of Food Choices

Our daily food choices wield a profound influence not only on immediate well-being but also on the long-term health of the gastrointestinal system.

The intricate interplay between the foods we consume and the gut's delicate ecosystem highlights the pivotal role of nutrition in maintaining a healthy and resilient digestive environment.

Microbial Balance:

Every meal shapes the composition of the gut microbiome. Opting for a diet rich in diverse, whole foods provides the necessary nutrients to sustain a balanced microbial community. These beneficial microbes play a crucial role in digestion, nutrient absorption, and immune system modulation.

Inflammation and Gut Integrity:

Certain food choices can either fuel or quell inflammation in the gut. Diets high in processed foods, artificial additives, and refined sugars may trigger inflammation, compromising the integrity of the intestinal lining. Conversely, anti-inflammatory foods, such as fatty fish, leafy greens, and berries, contribute to a healthier gut environment.

Impact on Tight Junctions:

Tight junctions between cells in the intestinal lining act as gatekeepers, regulating the passage of substances. Nutrient-dense foods, especially those rich in fiber, support the maintenance of these tight junctions, preventing the onset of increased intestinal permeability.

Gut-Brain Axis:

Emerging research emphasizes the intricate connection between the gut and the brain. Food choices can influence mental well-being through this gut-brain axis. Probiotic-rich foods, for example, may contribute to mood regulation and cognitive function.

Immune System Modulation:

The foods we choose to consume directly impact the functioning of the immune system. A diet abundant in vitamins, minerals, and antioxidants supports immune resilience, helping defend against infections and prevent inflammatory responses that could compromise gut health.

Common Dietary Triggers of Leaky Gut

The connection between diet and the development of a leaky gut underscores the significance of making informed dietary choices to support gastrointestinal health. Several common dietary triggers have been identified as potential contributors to increased intestinal permeability:

Gluten-Containing Grains:

Gluten, a protein found in wheat, barley, and rye, has been implicated in the disruption of tight junctions in susceptible individuals. For those with gluten sensitivity or celiac disease, the consumption of gluten-containing grains can lead to inflammation and compromise the integrity of the gut lining.

Dairy Products:

Certain proteins found in dairy, particularly casein and whey, may pose challenges for individuals with sensitivities. In some cases, dairy consumption has been associated with inflammation and increased gut permeability.

Refined Sugars:

Diets high in refined sugars and processed foods can negatively impact the gut microbiome. The proliferation of harmful bacteria at the expense of beneficial microbes may contribute to dysbiosis and compromise the gut barrier.

Processed Foods and Additives:

Highly processed foods often contain artificial additives, preservatives, and emulsifiers.

These substances may disrupt the balance of the gut microbiome and trigger inflammation, potentially contributing to increased intestinal permeability.

Excessive Alcohol Consumption:

Chronic and excessive alcohol intake has been linked to gut dysbiosis and increased intestinal permeability.

Alcohol can directly damage the cells lining the gut and impair their ability to form a protective barrier.

Artificial Sweeteners:

Some studies suggest a potential link between artificial sweeteners and alterations in gut bacteria, which could influence gut health. While more research is needed, limiting the consumption of artificial sweeteners is a cautious approach.

Recognizing and minimizing the impact of these common dietary triggers can be instrumental in preventing or managing leaky gut. Personalized dietary adjustments, guided by individual sensitivities and health considerations, contribute to a gut-friendly approach to nutrition and overall well-being.

Diagnosis and Treatment Options for Leaky Gut

Diagnosing and addressing a leaky gut involves a comprehensive approach that considers both symptoms and underlying factors contributing to increased intestinal permeability.

While there isn't a single diagnostic test exclusively for leaky gut, healthcare professionals employ a variety of methods to assess and address this condition.

- **Diagnosis:**

Symptom Assessment:

A thorough evaluation of symptoms, including digestive issues, fatigue, and inflammation, provides crucial initial insights. Identifying patterns and the duration of symptoms aids in the diagnostic process.

Blood Tests:

Elevated levels of certain antibodies or markers of inflammation in the blood may suggest gut dysfunction. However, these markers are not specific to leaky gut, necessitating a comprehensive analysis.

Lactulose-Mannitol Test:

This non-invasive test involves consuming a solution containing lactulose and mannitol, followed by measuring their levels in urine. Elevated lactulose levels relative to mannitol may indicate increased intestinal permeability.

Endoscopic Procedures:

In some cases, endoscopic examinations, such as a colonoscopy or upper endoscopy, may be performed to assess the condition of the intestinal lining directly.

- **Treatment Options:**

Dietary Modifications:

Eliminating or reducing common dietary triggers, such as gluten, dairy, and refined sugars, can help alleviate symptoms and support gut healing.

Nutritional Supplements:

Supplements like probiotics, prebiotics, and nutrients that promote gut health, such as glutamine and zinc, may be recommended to restore microbial balance and enhance intestinal barrier function.

Anti-Inflammatory Approaches:

Incorporating anti-inflammatory foods and lifestyle practices, such as omega-3 fatty acids and stress management, can help mitigate inflammation and promote gut healing.

Medication:

In certain cases, medications such as anti-inflammatory drugs or those addressing specific underlying conditions may be prescribed to manage symptoms and contribute to gut recovery.

Lifestyle Changes:

Stress reduction, regular exercise, and adequate sleep play integral roles in supporting overall health and may positively impact gut function.

As leaky gut is a multifaceted condition, a personalized and holistic approach to diagnosis and treatment, guided by healthcare professionals, is essential for addressing its complexities and promoting sustained gut health.

Lifestyle Changes for Managing Leaky Gut

Addressing a leaky gut involves not only dietary modifications but also comprehensive lifestyle changes that support gut health and overall well-being. These lifestyle adjustments are instrumental in reducing inflammation, promoting a balanced gut microbiome, and enhancing the integrity of the intestinal barrier.

Stress Management:

Chronic stress can significantly impact gut health by triggering inflammation and compromising the immune system. Incorporating stress-reducing practices such as mindfulness meditation, deep breathing exercises, and yoga can foster a more resilient response to stressors.

Adequate Sleep:

Quality sleep is essential for the repair and regeneration of the body, including the gut lining. Establishing consistent sleep patterns supports overall health and contributes to the optimal functioning of the gastrointestinal tract.

Regular Exercise:

Physical activity has been linked to a more diverse and balanced gut microbiome. Engaging in regular exercise not only supports overall health but also positively influences gut function and may contribute to a reduction in inflammation.

Hydration:

Maintaining adequate hydration is crucial for digestive health.

Water helps transport nutrients, supports the mucosal lining of the intestines, and aids in the elimination of waste. Optimal hydration contributes to a healthier gut environment.

Limiting Toxin Exposure:

Environmental toxins can impact gut health. Minimizing exposure to pollutants, pesticides, and unnecessary chemicals in household products can reduce the burden on the gut and support its healing.

Avoiding Overuse of Medications:

Certain medications, such as antibiotics and nonsteroidal anti-inflammatory drugs (NSAIDs), can disrupt the balance of the gut microbiome. When possible, limiting the unnecessary use of these medications supports a healthier gut environment.

Mindful Eating:

Eating in a relaxed environment, chewing food thoroughly, and savoring meals can contribute to better digestion. Mindful eating practices may help reduce stress on the digestive system and support gut health.

CHAPTER THREE

1. Probiotic Parfait

Ingredients:

1 cup Greek yogurt (probiotic-rich)

1/2 cup mixed berries

2 tablespoons chia seeds

1 tablespoon honey or maple syrup

Instructions:

In a bowl or glass, layer Greek yogurt.

Add a layer of mixed berries.

Sprinkle chia seeds on top.

Drizzle honey or maple syrup for sweetness.

Repeat layers as desired.

Preparation Time: 5 minutes

2. Turmeric Ginger Smoothie Bowl

Ingredients:

1 frozen banana

1/2 teaspoon turmeric powder

1 teaspoon fresh ginger, grated

1 cup spinach

1/2 cup almond milk

Toppings: sliced almonds, chia seeds

Instructions:

Blend frozen banana, turmeric, ginger, spinach, and almond milk until smooth.

Pour into a bowl.

Top with sliced almonds and chia seeds.

Preparation Time: 7 minutes

3. Quinoa Breakfast Bowl

Ingredients:

1/2 cup cooked quinoa

1/4 cup coconut milk

1/2 banana, sliced

1 tablespoon almond butter

1 tablespoon hemp seeds

Instructions:

Combine cooked quinoa and coconut milk in a bowl.

Top with banana slices.

Drizzle almond butter.

Sprinkle hemp seeds on top.

Preparation Time: 10 minutes

4. Egg and Avocado Toast

Ingredients:

2 slices whole-grain bread

2 eggs

1/2 avocado, sliced

Salt and pepper to taste

Instructions:

Toast the whole-grain bread.

Cook eggs as desired (poached, fried, or scrambled).

Place eggs on the toast.

Top with sliced avocado.

Season with salt and pepper.

Preparation Time: 15 minutes

5. Chia Seed Pudding

Ingredients:

3 tablespoons chia seeds

1 cup almond milk

1/2 teaspoon vanilla extract

Fresh berries for topping

Instructions:

Mix chia seeds, almond milk, and vanilla extract in a jar.

Refrigerate overnight or for at least 4 hours.

Top with fresh berries before serving.

Preparation Time: 5 minutes (+ chilling time)

6. Sweet Potato and Spinach Omelette

Ingredients:

2 eggs

1/2 cup cooked sweet potato, diced

Handful of fresh spinach

1 tablespoon olive oil

Salt and pepper to taste

Instructions:

Whisk eggs in a bowl.

In a pan, sauté spinach and sweet potato in olive oil until spinach wilts.

Pour whisked eggs over the vegetables.

Cook until eggs are set.

Season with salt and pepper.

Preparation Time: 12 minutes

7. Coconut Yogurt and Fruit Bowl

Ingredients:

1 cup coconut yogurt

1/2 cup granola (gluten-free if needed)

1/2 cup mixed tropical fruits (pineapple, mango, kiwi)

Instructions:

Spoon coconut yogurt into a bowl.

Top with granola.

Add mixed tropical fruits.

Preparation Time: 5 minutes

8. Green Detox Smoothie

Ingredients:

1 cup kale

1/2 cucumber, peeled

1/2 green apple, cored

1/2 lemon, juiced

1 cup coconut water

Ice cubes (optional)

Instructions:

Blend kale, cucumber, green apple, lemon juice, and coconut water until smooth.

Add ice cubes if desired.

Preparation Time: 8 minutes

9. Buckwheat Pancakes

Ingredients:

1/2 cup buckwheat flour

1/2 cup almond milk

1 egg

1/2 teaspoon baking powder

1 tablespoon coconut oil

Fresh berries for topping

Instructions:

Mix buckwheat flour, almond milk, egg, and baking powder in a bowl.

Heat coconut oil in a pan.

Pour batter into the pan to make pancakes.

Cook until bubbles form, then flip.

Top with fresh berries.

Preparation Time: 15 minutes

10. Mango Coconut Chia Pudding

Ingredients:

3 tablespoons chia seeds

1 cup coconut milk

1/2 cup fresh mango, diced

1 tablespoon shredded coconut

Instructions:

Mix chia seeds and coconut milk in a jar.

Refrigerate for at least 4 hours or overnight.

Top with fresh mango and shredded coconut before serving.

Preparation Time: 5 minutes (+ chilling time)

Healthy Lunch Leaky Guts Recipes

1. Quinoa and Vegetable Buddha Bowl:

Ingredients:

Cooked quinoa

Mixed vegetables (broccoli, bell peppers, carrots)

Avocado slices

Chickpeas (roasted)

Olive oil, lemon juice, and herbs for dressing

Instructions:

Mix cooked quinoa with roasted chickpeas and sautéed vegetables.

Top with avocado slices.

Drizzle with olive oil, lemon juice, and your favorite herbs.

Preparation Time: 20 minutes

2. Salmon and Spinach Salad:

Ingredients:

Grilled salmon fillet

Fresh spinach leaves

Cherry tomatoes

Cucumber slices

Avocado

Olive oil and balsamic vinaigrette

Instructions:

Arrange spinach on a plate, top with grilled salmon, and add vegetables.

Drizzle with olive oil and balsamic vinaigrette.

Preparation Time: 15 minutes

3. Turmeric Chickpea Stew:

Ingredients:

Chickpeas (canned or cooked)

Turmeric powder

Coconut milk

Spinach

Garlic and onion

Vegetable broth

Instructions:

Sauté garlic and onion, add chickpeas, turmeric, and vegetable broth.

Simmer until chickpeas are tender, then add coconut milk and spinach.

Preparation Time: 30 minutes

4. Zucchini Noodles with Pesto:

Ingredients:

Zucchini noodles

Cherry tomatoes

Pesto sauce (homemade or store-bought)

Pine nuts for garnish

Instructions:

Spiralize zucchini into noodles and toss with pesto.

Add cherry tomatoes and garnish with pine nuts.

Preparation Time: 15 minutes

5. Miso Soup with Tofu and Seaweed:

Ingredients:

Miso paste

Tofu cubes

Wakame seaweed

Green onions

Vegetable broth

Instructions:

Dissolve miso paste in vegetable broth.

Add tofu, seaweed, and green onions. Simmer until heated through.

Preparation Time: 20 minutes

6. Mediterranean Quinoa Salad:

Ingredients:

Cooked quinoa

Cherry tomatoes

Cucumber

Kalamata olives

Feta cheese

Olive oil and lemon dressing

Instructions:

Mix quinoa with chopped vegetables, olives, and feta.

Drizzle with olive oil and lemon dressing.

Preparation Time: 15 minutes

7. Ginger-Turmeric Chicken Stir-Fry:

Ingredients:

Chicken breast strips

Broccoli florets

Bell peppers

Ginger and turmeric

Tamari sauce

Sesame oil

Instructions:

Sauté chicken with ginger and turmeric.

Add vegetables, tamari sauce, and finish with a drizzle of sesame oil.

Preparation Time: 25 minutes

8. Sweet Potato and Lentil Curry:

Ingredients:

Sweet potatoes (diced)

Lentils

Coconut milk

Curry spices (cumin, coriander, turmeric)

Spinach

Instructions:

Cook lentils and sweet potatoes in coconut milk with curry spices.

Add spinach and simmer until wilted.

Preparation Time: 30 minutes

9. Avocado and Chickpea Wrap:

Ingredients:

Whole-grain wraps

Mashed avocado

Chickpeas (mashed)

Shredded carrots

Leafy greens

Hummus

Instructions:

Spread mashed avocado on wraps, add chickpeas, carrots, greens, and a dollop of hummus.

Roll and enjoy.

Preparation Time: 15 minutes

10. Roasted Vegetable Quiche:

Ingredients:

Whole-grain pie crust

Eggs

Mixed roasted vegetables (zucchini, bell peppers, tomatoes)

Feta cheese

Herbs (rosemary, thyme)

Instructions:

Whisk eggs and pour into the pie crust.

Add roasted vegetables, feta, and herbs.

Bake until the quiche is set.

Preparation Time: 40 minutes (including roasting time)

Healthy Dinner Leaky Guts Recipes

1. Quinoa and Vegetable Stir-Fry

Ingredients:

1 cup quinoa

Mixed vegetables (bell peppers, broccoli, carrots)

Tofu or chicken (optional)

Soy sauce

Olive oil

Garlic, minced

Ginger, grated

Instructions:

Cook quinoa according to package instructions.

In a pan, sauté garlic and ginger in olive oil.

Add mixed vegetables (and protein, if using) and stir-fry until tender.

Mix in cooked quinoa and soy sauce.

Serve hot.

Preparation Time: 25 minutes

2. Salmon and Asparagus Foil Pack

Ingredients:

Salmon fillets

Asparagus spears

Lemon slices

Olive oil

Garlic powder

Dill, chopped

Salt and pepper

Instructions:

Preheat the oven to 400°F (200°C).

Place salmon fillets on a foil sheet.

Arrange asparagus around the salmon.

Drizzle with olive oil, sprinkle with garlic powder, dill, salt, and pepper.

Place lemon slices on top.

Seal the foil and bake for 20 minutes.

Preparation Time: 30 minutes

3. Sweet Potato and Chickpea Curry

Ingredients:

Sweet potatoes, diced

Chickpeas, cooked

Coconut milk

Curry powder

Onion, chopped

Garlic, minced

Ginger, grated

Spinach leaves

Instructions:

Sauté onion, garlic, and ginger in a pot.

Add diced sweet potatoes and cook until slightly tender.

Stir in chickpeas, curry powder, and coconut milk.

Simmer until sweet potatoes are fully cooked.

Add spinach and cook until wilted.

Preparation Time: 40 minutes

4. Turkey and Vegetable Lettuce Wraps

Ingredients:

Ground turkey

Lettuce leaves

Bell peppers, diced

Carrots, shredded

Soy sauce

Sesame oil

Garlic, minced

Green onions, chopped

Instructions:

Cook ground turkey in a pan until browned.

Add garlic, bell peppers, and carrots.

Stir in soy sauce and sesame oil.

Spoon the mixture into lettuce leaves.

Garnish with green onions.

Preparation Time: 25 minutes

5. Mediterranean Quinoa Salad

Ingredients:

Quinoa, cooked

Cherry tomatoes, halved

Cucumber, diced

Kalamata olives, sliced

Feta cheese, crumbled

Red onion, finely chopped

Olive oil

Lemon juice

Fresh oregano, chopped

Instructions:

Combine quinoa, cherry tomatoes, cucumber, olives, feta, and red onion in a bowl.

In a separate bowl, whisk together olive oil, lemon juice, and oregano.

Toss the quinoa mixture with the dressing.

Chill before serving.

Preparation Time: 20 minutes

6. Chicken and Vegetable Skewers

Ingredients:

Chicken breast, cubed

Bell peppers, cut into chunks

Zucchini, sliced

Cherry tomatoes

Olive oil

Garlic powder

Paprika

Lemon juice

Instructions:

Preheat the grill or oven.

Thread chicken, bell peppers, zucchini, and tomatoes onto skewers.

Mix olive oil, garlic powder, paprika, and lemon juice.

Brush skewers with the mixture.

Grill or bake until chicken is cooked through.

Preparation Time: 30 minutes

7. Spinach and Mushroom Quiche

Ingredients:

Quiche crust (store-bought or homemade)

Eggs

Spinach, chopped

Mushrooms, sliced

Feta cheese

Milk or alternative

Nutmeg

Salt and pepper

Instructions:

Preheat the oven to 375°F (190°C).

In a bowl, whisk eggs, milk, nutmeg, salt, and pepper.

Arrange spinach, mushrooms, and feta on the quiche crust.

Pour the egg mixture over the ingredients.

Bake for 35-40 minutes.

Preparation Time: 50 minutes

8. Lentil and Vegetable Soup

Ingredients:

Lentils, rinsed

Carrots, diced

Celery, chopped

Onion, diced

Garlic, minced

Vegetable broth

Tomato paste

Cumin

Turmeric

Paprika

Bay leaves

Instructions:

In a pot, sauté onion and garlic until softened.

Add lentils, carrots, celery, and tomato paste.

Pour in vegetable broth and add cumin, turmeric, paprika, and bay leaves.

Simmer until lentils and vegetables are tender.

Preparation Time: 45 minutes

9. Shrimp and Avocado Salad

Ingredients:

Shrimp, cooked and peeled

Mixed salad greens

Avocado, sliced

Cherry tomatoes, halved

Red onion, thinly sliced

Cilantro, chopped

Olive oil

Lime juice

Salt and pepper

Instructions:

Arrange salad greens on plates.

Top with shrimp, avocado, tomatoes, red onion, and cilantro.

Whisk together olive oil, lime juice, salt, and pepper.

Drizzle the dressing over the salad.

Preparation Time: 15 minutes

10. Baked Cod with Lemon and Herbs

Ingredients:

Cod fillets

Lemon slices

Fresh herbs (parsley, dill, thyme)

Olive oil

Garlic, minced

Salt and pepper

Instructions:

Preheat the oven to 375°F (190°C).

Place cod fillets in a baking dish.

Drizzle with olive oil, sprinkle with minced garlic, salt, and pepper.

Top with lemon slices and fresh herbs.

Bake for 15-20 minutes or until the fish flakes easily.

Preparation Time: 25 minutes

Healthy Snack Leaky Guts Recipes

1. Turmeric Roasted Chickpeas

Ingredients:

1 can (15 oz) chickpeas, drained and rinsed

1 tablespoon olive oil

1 teaspoon turmeric

1/2 teaspoon cumin

Salt and pepper to taste

Instructions:

Preheat the oven to 400°F (200°C).

Pat the chickpeas dry with a paper towel.

Toss chickpeas in olive oil, turmeric, cumin, salt, and pepper.

Spread them on a baking sheet and bake for 25-30 minutes, or until golden and crispy.

Preparation Time: 35 minutes

2. Avocado and Salmon Nori Rolls

Ingredients:

Nori sheets

1 ripe avocado, sliced

Smoked salmon slices

Cucumber strips

Sesame seeds for garnish

Instructions:

Place a nori sheet on a bamboo sushi rolling mat.

Spread avocado slices, smoked salmon, and cucumber strips.

Roll tightly and slice into bite-sized pieces.

Sprinkle with sesame seeds.

Preparation Time: 15 minutes

3. Zucchini Noodle Salad with Pesto

Ingredients:

Zucchini noodles

Cherry tomatoes, halved

1/4 cup pine nuts

Fresh basil leaves

Olive oil, lemon juice, salt, and pepper

Instructions:

Toss zucchini noodles, cherry tomatoes, and pine nuts in a bowl.

In a blender, blend fresh basil, olive oil, lemon juice, salt, and pepper to make pesto.

Drizzle pesto over the salad and toss.

Preparation Time: 20 minutes

4. Sweet Potato and Kale Chips

Ingredients:

Sweet potatoes, thinly sliced

Kale leaves, stems removed

Olive oil

Sea salt

Instructions:

Preheat the oven to 375°F (190°C).

Toss sweet potato slices and kale with olive oil.

Spread on baking sheets, sprinkle with sea salt, and bake for 15-20 minutes.

Preparation Time: 30 minutes

5. Coconut Yogurt Parfait

Ingredients:

Coconut yogurt

Berries (blueberries, strawberries)

Almond slices

Chia seeds

Instructions:

In a glass, layer coconut yogurt, berries, almond slices, and chia seeds.

Repeat layers.

Top with additional berries.

Preparation Time: 10 minutes

6. Protein-Packed Energy Bites

Ingredients:

1 cup rolled oats

1/2 cup almond butter

1/4 cup honey

1/4 cup chia seeds

1/4 cup dark chocolate chips

Instructions:

Mix rolled oats, almond butter, honey, chia seeds, and chocolate chips in a bowl.

Form into bite-sized balls and refrigerate for at least 30 minutes.

Preparation Time: 15 minutes

7. Cucumber Hummus Boats

Ingredients:

Cucumbers, halved and seeds removed

Hummus

Cherry tomatoes, sliced

Fresh dill for garnish

Instructions:

Fill cucumber halves with hummus.

Top with cherry tomato slices and garnish with fresh dill.

Preparation Time: 10 minutes

8. Almond and Coconut Protein Bars

Ingredients:

1 cup almonds

1/2 cup shredded coconut

1/4 cup protein powder

1/4 cup almond butter

2 tablespoons honey

Instructions:

Blend almonds and shredded coconut in a food processor.

Add protein powder, almond butter, and honey. Blend until combined.

Press into a pan and refrigerate for 1 hour. Cut into bars.

Preparation Time: 15 minutes

9. Spinach and Artichoke Dip with Veggie Sticks

Ingredients:

1 cup steamed spinach

1/2 cup artichoke hearts, chopped

1/2 cup Greek yogurt

1/4 cup grated Parmesan cheese

Carrot and cucumber sticks for dipping

Instructions:

Mix steamed spinach, chopped artichoke hearts, Greek yogurt, and Parmesan cheese.

Serve with carrot and cucumber sticks.

Preparation Time: 20 minutes

10. Blueberry Almond Smoothie Bowl

Ingredients:

1 cup frozen blueberries

1 banana

1/2 cup almond milk

Toppings: sliced almonds, chia seeds, fresh blueberries

Instructions:

Blend frozen blueberries, banana, and almond milk until smooth.

Pour into a bowl and top with sliced almonds, chia seeds, and fresh blueberries.

Preparation Time: 5 minutes

CONCLUSION

Embarking on a journey toward digestive wellness through the pages of this Leaky Gut Cookbook has been akin to savoring the chapters of a transformative culinary adventure. In the vibrant tapestry of recipes and insights, we've explored the delicate interplay between nutrition, lifestyle, and the intricate ecosystem that is the gut.

As the flavors and aromas of gut-friendly ingredients infused our kitchens, we've come to appreciate the profound impact of mindful food choices on the health of our intestinal terrain. The recipes within these pages not only tantalize the taste buds but serve as a roadmap, guiding us towards a harmonious relationship with our digestive systems.

Beyond the realm of recipes, we've uncovered the significance of lifestyle adjustments—embracing stress-soothing practices, prioritizing restful sleep, and incorporating joyful movement into our days.

This holistic approach acknowledges that true gut health is a symphony, where every ingredient, every lifestyle choice, contributes to the harmonious melody of well-being.

As we conclude this culinary odyssey, let us carry forward the lessons learned, savoring not just the flavors but the wisdom ingrained in each dish.

May these recipes and insights empower us to make informed choices, fostering a gut environment that is resilient, vibrant, and a cornerstone of our overall vitality.

In the kitchen and beyond, may the Leaky Gut Cookbook inspire a lifelong commitment to digestive wellness, reminding us that the journey to a healthier gut is not just a destination but a continuous celebration of the nourishing connection between what we eat and how we live.